The After-Shift Reset Guide for Night-Shift Clinicians

10-Minute Wind-Down Routines, Sleep-Support Habits, and Nervous-System Calming Tools for Hospital and EMS Teams

Disclaimer

By reading or using this guide, you agree to the terms of this disclaimer. If you do not accept these terms, discontinue use.

This guide is for informational and educational purposes only. It is not professional advice of any kind, including but not limited to financial, legal, business, psychological, or career counseling. The author is not a licensed professional in these fields, and reading this guide does not create any client, advisory, or professional relationship.

You should consult qualified professionals regarding any decisions related to your personal, financial, legal, business, or psychological situation. Do not treat the content of this guide as a substitute for professional guidance.

The information provided is based on research and personal interpretation. While efforts were made to ensure accuracy, the author and publisher make no guarantees or warranties regarding completeness, reliability, or suitability of the material. You assume full responsibility for how you choose to use this information. To the fullest extent permitted by law, the author and publisher disclaim all liability for any loss, damage, or consequences arising from your reliance on this guide.

No specific results, achievements, or outcomes are promised or implied. Individual experiences will vary.

Any tools, brand names, concepts, or examples referenced are the property of their respective owners and are used for informational purposes only. Their inclusion does not imply endorsement. Any individuals appearing in cover or promotional images are stock models used under appropriate licenses.

Table of Contents

Introduction: Resetting After the Night Shift, Why It Matters for You Now

Night-shift clinicians and EMS professionals face a unique set of challenges that set your experience apart from daytime peers. You're managing patient needs or acute incidents at hours when your body craves rest, often navigating unpredictable emergencies on little sleep or while your circadian clock signals it's time for bed. This relentless schedule brings more than simple tiredness. It can lead to a deep, physical and mental fatigue, fragmented sleep, and stress that lingers long after your shift ends. Over time, these pressures may escalate into burnout or chronic health issues if left unchecked.

This guide is designed with your real-life demands in mind. The goal isn't to add more complexity to your day, but to provide clear, actionable tools you can deploy immediately after a shift. You'll learn how to implement fast-acting routines that bring down stress quickly, establish sleep habits that support healthy recovery, calm your nervous system with science-backed approaches, and build a practical defense against long-term exhaustion. Every recommendation considers the urgency and reality of post-shift life in clinical or high-stress environments. By focusing on what you can control after your shift ends, you'll make measurable improvements in how you recover and ultimately in your ability to continue working safely and effectively.

There are a few important boundaries to clarify before you dive in. This guide is not a handbook for on-shift performance strategies. It doesn't address advanced psychiatric conditions or delve into complex pharmacology. If you require a deeper clinical intervention, or have a diagnosed mental health condition needing medical management, use these tools as supportive additions only with guidance from your healthcare provider. The focus here is strictly on practical, evidence-based resets you can use after your shift, habits and interventions proven to help you recover, decompress, and prevent the build-up of stress-related damage.

You're in the right place if you're a frontline hospital worker, EMS professional, or clinician routinely working nights or variable shifts. This resource is specifically built for you, someone who needs recovery strategies that are fast, streamlined, and rooted in clinical evidence. It's not aimed at office-based staff, daytime workers, or those outside the field. Each chapter targets the realities of night-shift healthcare: physical drag, mental fog, and the struggle to "switch off" when the rest of the world is just waking up.

How should you use this guide? The chapters are modular. If there's a particular area that's causing the most strain e.g., persistent hyperarousal, poor sleep, physical tension, or difficulty winding down, feel free to jump to that section first and implement the proposed solution immediately. If you want a comprehensive approach, move through the guide sequentially to build a personalized reset system step-by-step. Either way, you're encouraged to experiment and adapt, choosing the methods that fit your own energy patterns, schedule, and environment.

Resetting after the night shift is not a luxury. It is a critical investment in your health, your cognitive performance, and your safety in a demanding profession. The actionable routines ahead are designed to fit the realities of your life now, so you can recover faster and protect your long-term well-being, shift after shift.

Chapter 1: The Science of Night-Shift Fatigue

Understanding the science behind night-shift fatigue is essential for hospital and EMS professionals who work against the body's natural clock. Working at night disrupts not only sleep schedules but also the deep-seated biological rhythms that regulate alertness and recovery. In this chapter, you'll see how circadian misalignment uniquely affects those in clinical and emergency settings, learn to spot the signs of persistent fatigue, and discover why "toughing it out" backfires. You'll also get direct tools for self-monitoring before fatigue becomes critical.

Sleep-Wake Cycle Disruption and Circadian Misalignment

Humans have an internal clock, your circadian rhythm, entrained by cues like daylight and regular sleep-wake times. For most, this clock primes the body to be awake and alert during the day, and to wind down at night. Night-shift work turns this pattern upside down.

In hospital and EMS environments, night-shifters move through bright, noisy settings while their brains are biologically scheduled for rest. Essential hormones such as melatonin (which signals sleepiness) and cortisol (which promotes alertness) are out of sync. As a result, you often feel a sluggish mental fog in the early morning, struggle to fall or stay asleep during the day, and find your body fighting the expectations of shift schedules. Even with blackout curtains or caffeine, your body's physiology pushes back, making full recovery challenging without deliberate strategies.

Checklist: Five Primary Symptoms of Chronic Shift-Induced Fatigue

Recognizing the onset of fatigue is the first step in preventing long-term consequences.

Here are the top five symptoms to watch for in yourself:

1. Persistent grogginess, even after what "should" be enough sleep and even on days off.
2. Frequent memory lapses or difficulty focusing, noticeable during simple tasks or patient handoffs.
3. Irritability and low mood that lingers past the end of your shift.
4. Increased physical clumsiness or slow reaction times.
5. Headaches, stomach upset, or mild dizziness recurring after multiple shifts.

Not every symptom points to a crisis, but a pattern, especially two or more symptoms lingering several days in a row, warrants careful attention.

Case Examples: What Happens When After-Shift Routines Fail

The risks tied to unaddressed after-shift fatigue are real. Consider these scenarios:

An overnight respiratory therapist, after three consecutive shifts, skips her usual cool-down to nap in her car with the radio on. She wakes, groggy, drives home, and misses a stop sign en route.

A paramedic, feeling wired and exhausted, forgoes winding down and immediately tries to nap in a brightly lit room at home. He wakes up mentally foggy and later at work struggles to recall a medication dosage, nearly administering the wrong amount.

A night ward nurse, unable to unplug after shift, endlessly scrolls her phone before bed, then struggles with racing thoughts and delayed sleep. The next evening, she forgets a key part of her PPE protocol during a code.

These examples underscore how neglected post-shift routines amplify mistakes, create safety risks, and set off a cycle of declining alertness across multiple shifts. In most clinical settings, fatigue isn't just personal. It becomes a systems issue.

Step-by-Step: Self-Identifying and Tracking Emerging Fatigue

To get ahead of fatigue, you need to build awareness. Self-monitoring with a fatigue log reveals early trends you might otherwise brush aside as "just a bad day." Here's a simple way to start:

- Pick a medium (notebook, phone app, or notes on your work device).
- After every shift, pause for two minutes to check in on the five core symptoms listed earlier.
- Log a quick note: Mark which symptoms you notice, rate their severity (mild, moderate, severe), and jot down any incidents or moments you felt "off."
- Track your sleep details: actual hours slept, disruptions, and quality ("restful" or "fragmented").
- End your log with one sentence summarizing post-shift recovery: "Felt focused after wind-down routine" or "Wired and unable to slow down," for example.

Aim to log for two weeks. Patterns will emerge—maybe fatigue spikes on certain shift sequences or worsens when you skip wind-down steps. This personal data strengthens your ability to course-correct early, before fatigue progresses to burnout.

Debunking the Most Common Misconceptions About "Powering Through"

In clinical environments, it's common to hear myths about handling night shifts. Here's what research and daily experience consistently prove wrong:

- ***Misconception 1***: "If I just push through, I'll adjust soon enough."

  Reality: Few people fully adapt to night shifts. Most remain biologically out of sync; fatigue accumulates, leading to chronic deficits in alertness and recovery.

- ***Misconception 2***: "Coffee or energy drinks make up for lost sleep."

  Reality: Stimulants may mask tiredness temporarily, but they do not restore lost attention, memory, or physical coordination. Overuse often worsens sleep problems post-shift.

- ***Misconception 3***: "Other people handle nights fine. If I can't, it's a personal weakness."

  Reality: Most night-shift workers, including seasoned staff, run into these same fatigue pitfalls. Problems signal the need for supportive habits—not a lack of willpower or skill.

- ***Misconception 4***: “Catching up on sleep later erases night-shift debt.”

  Reality: “Banking” sleep doesn’t undo the effects of circadian rhythm disruption or immediately restore cognitive performance. Consistency in after-shift recovery is far more protective.

- ***Misconception 5***: “It’s normal to feel this exhausted—it’s just part of the job.”

  Reality: While night shifts are demanding, deep, persistent fatigue is not something to normalize. Ongoing impairment means underlying routines and support systems need adjusting.

Bringing These Principles Forward

Grasping the science and patterns behind night-shift fatigue arms you with an essential baseline for intervention. Recognizing your own early warning signs, logging real after-shift experiences, and rejecting harmful myths put you back in control. The next step is to leverage rapid, evidence-based wind-down strategies that set the foundation for quality rest and safe re-entry on your next shift.

Chapter 2: The 10-Minute Wind-Down: Why It's Non-Negotiable

Shifting gears from the clinical intensity of night work to recovery mode is more than a luxury. It's a biological necessity. Now that you've seen how deep the impact of shift fatigue runs, it's time to talk about the single most actionable antidote available: the 10-minute wind-down. This isn't an optional perk or a vague wellness tip. It's a brief but critical window where you intentionally reset your nervous system and set the stage for real rest.

Why decompression is urgent: the neurobiology of the shift wind-down

Clinical work at night keeps your sympathetic nervous system fired up. Long after you clock out, stress hormones like cortisol and adrenaline remain high. Data consistently show that after a demanding shift, cortisol levels can remain elevated for up to an hour, sometimes more, especially when the transition home is abrupt or stressful. In this state, your body is trapped in "work mode": muscles tense, heart rate elevated, mind racing.

What you need immediately post-shift is a rapid signal switch, from sympathetic arousal to parasympathetic recovery. This is the phase when your heart rate slows, your digestion resumes, and the body preps for true relaxation and sleep. Research on shift workers highlights that even just 10 minutes of intentional calming—via breathwork, gentle movement, or sensory cues—can measurably decrease cortisol and initiate

parasympathetic rebound. The bottom line: without this reset, your body and mind remain in a low-grade state of emergency, which drags out fatigue and impairs recovery.

The basic 10-minute wind-down protocol

Clinicians need a routine that is automatic, portable, and non-intrusive. You have limited time and unpredictable environments at shift end. The following template can be adapted for a break room, your car, or at home, and focuses on the minimum viable steps for nervous system reset:

1. Find as much quiet and separation as possible. If you're sharing a break room, use noise-cancelling headphones or play calming ambient noise. Dim any harsh lighting if you can.
2. Sit comfortably or recline, keeping your spine supported.
3. Close your eyes or soften your gaze. Take three slow, deliberate breaths: inhale through your nose for a count of four, exhale gently for six.

4. Scan your body for tension (jaw, shoulders, back). As you exhale, imagine letting the weight drop away. Brief stretching here, even rolling your shoulders or neck, can help.
5. If safe and private, try three to five minutes of guided breathwork or a short relaxation audio clip (preloaded on your phone to avoid distractions).
6. For the final few minutes, focus on a calming rhythm. This might be slow breathing, listening to mellow music, or, if you're at home, standing by a darkened window for a few quiet moments.

If needed, adapt the steps to fit your situation. In your car, simply recline the seat slightly, limit input from your phone, and focus on your breath for several minutes before driving home. At home, use this protocol as soon as you come in, before checking messages or starting chores.

How to choose between a quick wind-down and a full-length reset

You won't always have bandwidth or time for a longer recovery routine, but a quick reset is non-negotiable when:

- Your mind is racing and your body feels "on edge."
- You have only 10-15 minutes before sleep or your commute.
- You notice mental fatigue but can still function safely.

Reserve full-length resets (30 minutes or more involving movement, shower, or extended meditation) for those times when you feel:

- Deep muscle exhaustion or emotional depletion lingering after brief wind-down.
- Physical signs like racing heart, GI discomfort, or residual tremor.
- You're heading directly into a sleep window and need to maximize rest depth.

A helpful rule: If you feel "wired but tired," do the 10-minute protocol. If you feel so depleted you're moving in slow motion, or can't disengage from work thoughts, consider a longer, more structured routine before sleep.

Top three wind-down sabotage pitfalls and how to avoid them

Many clinicians unintentionally trip themselves up during wind-down. Here are the most common mistakes:

- Immediate phone or screen use. Checking email, news, or messages signals your brain to stay alert, blocking your nervous system from downshifting. Delay screens until your wind-down is finished.
- Ruminating over shift details. Mentally rehashing errors or stressful moments keeps your stress

chemistry high. If your mind starts racing, focus back on your breath or the physical cues in your body.

- Skipping the routine "just this once." Telling yourself you're too tired or busy to decompress quickly snowballs into habit loss. Even a five-minute placeholder is better than nothing. Consistency signals your system that it's time to shift gears.

Quick metrics for measuring wind-down effectiveness

You don't need lab results or elaborate trackers to know if your wind-down is working. Use these simple self-checks immediately after your routine:

- ***Heart rate***: Noticeable drop, or at least no palpitations or rapid beats.
- ***Muscle and jaw tension***: Marked softening, less clenching, or an easier relaxed posture.
- ***Mental state***: Racing thoughts quieted or replaced by a sense of "letting go"; intrusive shift details fade.
- ***Breathing***: Naturally deeper or slower with less effort.

Optionally, rate these on a 1–5 scale (1 = highly stressed/tight, 5 = noticeably relaxed).

Tracking your subjective ratings for a week or two will reveal patterns and highlight when you need to adjust your routine.

A targeted wind-down does more than just feel good. It creates a measurable shift in your readiness for true rest. As you practice and refine your 10-minute routine, you'll notice clearer transitions from work to recovery, fewer after-shift crashes, and a more reliable entry into sleep. The next chapter will guide you in personalizing this reset for your commute and home environment, ensuring your post-shift decompression fits your real-world workflow.

Chapter 3: Building Your Personalized After-Shift Reset

No two clinicians will have identical after-shift needs, and the key to reliable recovery is creating a reset plan that respects your unique fatigue patterns, commute, and living situation. Building a personalized reset means more than doing what's "recommended." It means mapping every step from the hospital door to your bed and actively shaping your decompression window. Here's how to turn your unpredictable post-shift slog into a smooth, supportive transition.

How to Map Your Commute and Home Environment for Optimal Decompression

Start by viewing your commute and arrival home as active ingredients in your reset, not just filler time between work and sleep. The aim is to smooth the transition and reduce the friction that keeps you "stuck in work mode."

1. First, map your commute. Identify potential trouble spots and opportunities for decompression:
    - Do you have a long drive or a short walk? Does public transport demand alertness, or can you "downshift" during the ride?
    - Are there overstimulating elements, like bright headlights, noisy traffic, or crowded trains? Or

do you have autonomy over your environment, such as playing calming music or using noise-canceling headphones?

- Is your arrival routine rushed, with lots of lights, family chatter, or digital distractions the moment you open the door, or are there quiet minutes before you need to interact?

2. Next, evaluate your home entry sequence. Are you greeted by clutter, a loud TV, notifications, or pets needing care? All of these become micro-barriers or micro-boosts depending on your approach. Think about simple tweaks:
    - Leaving a dim lamp on instead of overhead lights.
    - Prepping blackout curtains or eye masks so they're ready.
    - Creating a dedicated surface for your work gear, so your brain gets a single, clear signal: shift over.

Small changes here can radically change how quickly your nervous system can power down. If you share your home, communicate your "reset window" to family or roommates, 10–30 minutes where you need minimal noise, questions, or requests.

Worksheet: Identify Your Three Highest-Yield Reset Habits

Not all decompression tactics carry equal weight. You want to prioritize "reset habits" that instantly deliver a big impact, both on your body and on your odds of successful sleep.

Run this quick worksheet (do it now or jot down your responses for later):

Recall the last five post-shift wind-downs you attempted. What single action gave you the most relief or reliably signaled, "The shift is over"?

- What are the top three things that, when skipped, leave you feeling wired or irritable for hours?
- Of all the relaxation or transition habits you've heard about, which feel realistic for you given your actual living conditions, time constraints, and personality?

From these responses, extract your three highest-yield reset habits. Common options include:

- ☐ Brief, slow walk (even just around the block or parking lot).
- ☐ Hot (or cool) shower right on arrival.
- ☐ Setting a sleep cue, like lavender spray, white noise, or blackout shades.
- ☐ Switching from scrubs/work gear to home clothes immediately.

☐ Using a short breathing exercise or mindfulness audio during the commute.

Keep your list visible for one week. See if these three habits work as "anchors" for your routine. Revise as needed—they should make your transition home measurably smoother.

Decision Tree: Customizing Routines by Energy Level and Sleep Window

Every shift ends differently. Sometimes you finish with enough adrenaline to run a marathon; other times, you're so wiped out that standing in the shower feels like too much.

A rigid routine is likely to fail, flexibility is smarter.

Use this quick decision framework:

<u>Assess your energy as you clock out:</u>

☐ Wired (racy mind, body buzzing, not sleepy)
☐ Depleted (heavy, foggy, barely alert)

Note your available sleep window before your next obligation:

☐ Ample (5+ hours)
☐ Tight (<4 hours)

Now:

- If Wired + Ample Window: Do a longer wind-down (10–20 minutes). Include a slow walk/stretch, extended shower, and intentional sleep cues.
- If Wired + Tight Window: Compress the essentials—pick one grounding technique (e.g., breathwork or home clothes change) and limit digital/device exposure.
- If Depleted + Ample Window: Prioritize immediate sleep cues (dark, cool room, low stimulation). Move directly from door to bed if possible, skipping optional steps.
- If Depleted + Tight Window: Do the absolute minimum needed for hygiene and comfort; set up an alarm and block all distractions. Consider a micro-reset (2–3 minutes) if skipping wind-down results in poor sleep.

Adapt routines daily. The right reset is the one you actually complete, not the theoretical "perfect" one.

Three Contrasting Clinician Reset Plans—and Their Outcomes

To put this in context, consider these sample reset plans:

1. ***Clinician 1***: Urban ICU nurse, 30-minute subway ride, two young children at home. Her top reset habits:
    - Noise-canceling headphones and guided body-scan meditation on the train.

- Text to family 5 minutes before home, cueing them to keep early mornings quiet.
- Quick hand-and-face wash, blackout curtains up immediately.
- ***Result***: Faster heart rate drop after shifts, smoother transition to sleep, fewer early morning disruptions.

2. ***Clinician 2***: Rural EMS worker, solo drive home after call-heavy night. Reset habits:
    - Calming playlist on car stereo during final 10 minutes.
    - Immediately removes work boots and uniform at the door.
    - Breathwork (4-7-8 breathing) for two cycles before bed.
    - Result: Reports shorter "wakeful" time before sleep onset; feels less tense upon waking.
    - Clinician 3: Hospital respiratory therapist, lives with roommate, short bicycle commute.
    - Rigid about two things:
    - Shower and podcast as soon as she gets in.
    - Eye mask and "do not disturb" sign on door; phone on silent.
    - ***Result***: Increased sleep duration, fewer roommate interruptions, easier time maintaining the reset on back-to-back shift blocks.

Each routine is tailored and may look simple, but the effect can be major. The shared success factor: consistency and honest adaptation to changing energy and home demands.

Troubleshooting: When Your Reset Is Interrupted or Derailed

Even well-designed routines break down. Kids wake early, your commute is delayed, or a mandatory after-shift meeting pops up. To avoid a total derailment:

- Have a "micro-reset" you can deploy anywhere. For example, 60 seconds of slow breathing while in the restroom or an elevator.
- If family or roommates interrupt, communicate boundaries in advance. Create a visual cue—a sign on the door, headphones in, or a scheduled "off duty" time.
- If your mind is spinning with work replay, don't force sleep. Jot down a quick "brain dump" in your notes app, then return to your sleep routine.
- If your schedule is upended (unexpected call-in, fire alarm, or event), pick up your routine at the next possible moment—in the car, shower, or even seated on your bed. Partial completion beats total abandonment.

A flexible reset plan doesn't fail at the first bump. It evolves, recognizing that even tiny rituals, done consistently, help send the signal: you are off the clock and moving toward genuine rest.

By customizing your after-shift reset, adapting its intensity, and troubleshooting setbacks, you’re designing a routine you can rely on. As you move into the next chapter, you’ll learn targeted tools, like breathwork, that further accelerate this critical transition.

Chapter 4: Breathwork Protocols for Rapid Nervous-System Calming

A smooth commute home sets the stage for effective recovery, but managing your body's stress response requires more than just changing your physical environment. Breathwork, simple, structured breathing exercises, is one of the fastest, most researched tools available for calming the nervous system. For clinicians coming off high-alert night shifts, these protocols can help transition from work-mode vigilance to a calmer state, improving your ability to fall asleep, think clearly, and recover for the next shift.

Evidence-backed overview of breathwork benefits for post-shift clinicians

The physiological link between breathing and nervous system regulation is well established. Shifts in respiratory pattern can rapidly influence your heart rate, blood pressure, and the delicate balance between 'fight-or-flight' (sympathetic) and 'rest-and-digest' (parasympathetic) states. Clinical studies show that slow, controlled breathing activates the vagus nerve—an essential switch for turning down excessive stress responses. Among hospital workers, nurses, and EMS professionals, research suggests that as little as five minutes of breath-controlled exercise reduces heart rate variability and self-reported anxiety. For night-shift clinicians, using breathwork immediately after a shift can:

- Lower circulating stress hormones (cortisol, adrenaline)
- Reduce mental rumination and muscle tension
- Speed up the transition toward sleep readiness

Reinforce the psychological boundary between work and off-duty time

The immediate feedback of breathwork is also appealing: most people notice a drop in heart rate and sense of urgency within just a few cycles.

Step-by-step instructions: Box breathing, 4-7-8, and extended exhale techniques

Let's cover three evidence-based breathing protocols that are practical for use at the end of your shift, wherever you are.

- ***Box Breathing*** (also called square breathing)
    1. Inhale slowly through your nose for 4 counts
    2. Hold your breath for 4 counts
    3. Exhale slowly through your mouth for 4 counts
    4. Hold with lungs empty for 4 counts

  Repeat 3–5 cycles (or longer as needed), keeping each phase equal in length. This method gently balances oxygen and carbon dioxide, stabilizing your heart rate and focus.

- ***4–7–8 Breathing***
    1. Inhale quietly through your nose for 4 counts
    2. Hold your breath for 7 counts
    3. Exhale audibly through your mouth for 8 counts

  Aim for four cycles. The extended hold and longer exhale increase relaxation and help downregulate nervous system overactivity. For beginners, you may start with shorter holds (e.g., 4–4–6) and work up.

- ***Extended Exhale Breathing***
    1. Inhale through your nose for 4–5 counts
    2. Exhale slowly for 6–8 counts (mouth or nose)

  No breath holds are required. Continue for 1–2 minutes. Prioritizing a longer exhale increases parasympathetic (rest-and-digest) activity, making this protocol fast-acting for acute anxiety or lingering adrenaline.

Choose a protocol that fits where you are: in your parked car, break room, or immediately after walking in the door.

Quick reference guide: Choosing the right protocol for your mood/disposition

Not every breathwork protocol feels the same, and your current state matters. Use this quick guide to match method to mood:

1. Wired, restless, or having trouble "shifting gears": Start with box breathing for 2–3 minutes. Its symmetry calms racing thoughts.
2. Feeling agitated, heart pounding, or coming off an adrenaline spike: 4–7–8 breathing harnesses longer exhales and holds to deepen relaxation.
3. Overwhelmed, anxious, or tense and can't settle: Extended exhale techniques work best when you need immediate reduction in arousal and no effortful holds.

If you feel sluggish or too fatigued, all three can be performed gently, slow the pace, shorten the holds, or do fewer cycles.

See what feels best and adjust as needed. The goal isn't to "master" the technique but to nudge your system toward calm.

Checklist: Signs you need to use breathwork vs. other tools

Not every post-shift challenge demands breathwork. Use this checklist to identify when it's likely to help, and when to consider another tool from your reset toolkit.

Use breathwork when you notice:

- ☐ Heart racing or palpitations as you sign out or head home
- ☐ Racing or looping thoughts about patients or clinical events

- ☐ Dread or tension as you approach your bed (can't turn off alertness)
- ☐ Physical symptoms like clenched jaw, tight chest, or shallow breathing
- ☐ Inability to transition from "task mode" to "recovery mode" despite leaving work
- ☐ Previous experience of wind-down routines taking too long to make an impact
- ☐ Consider other tools (e.g., movement, environment adjustment, brief social check-in) when breathing exercises cause discomfort, dizziness, or increased agitation
- ☐ You feel physically sluggish but not mentally activated
- ☐ Your main barrier to sleep is pain, hunger, or environmental factors
- ☐ Pausing for two minutes to check in with these signs helps clarify your next best step.

Cautions: When to avoid or modify breath-focused exercises (respiratory considerations)

Breathwork is generally safe for most healthy adults, but there are situations where you should proceed cautiously or skip these techniques:

If you have chronic respiratory conditions (asthma, COPD, recent respiratory infection): Use only gentle, short-duration protocols. Stop if you experience shortness of breath, coughing, or chest tightness.

Anyone prone to hyperventilation, panic attacks, or fainting should start with minimal cycles and avoid long breath holds.

Pregnant clinicians, or those with recent thoracic surgery, should consult a medical provider before starting new breathing routines.

Never practice breathwork while operating a vehicle or machinery, save it for when you're fully stationary.

If you feel dizzy, nauseated, or unusually anxious during breathwork, stop immediately and return to your usual breathing. You can return to breathwork later or choose an alternative wind-down strategy from your reset plan.

Bringing breathwork into your post-shift toolkit doesn't require perfection, just consistency and a willingness to pause. The more familiar these patterns become, the faster you'll feel their nervous-system-calming effects. In the next section, you'll learn how to combine breathwork with targeted micro-movement for an even more thorough after-shift recovery.

Chapter 5: Micro-Movement: Targeted Physical Reset in Under 10 Minutes

Physical movement is often the missing ingredient in a post-shift reset. While breathwork effectively guides your mind toward calm, gentle physical activity helps the body complete its transition out of high-alert mode. After a demanding night, your system can remain on edge, adrenaline lingering, muscles tight, nerves firing. Even brief, low-intensity movement acts as a reset switch, targeting those stress signals at their source.

How Micro-Movements Calm the Nervous System

Gentle movement works on several levels. First, slow stretching or easy walking stimulates circulation, clearing away metabolic byproducts that build up after hours on your feet, or worse, in tense, static postures. These movements send feedback to your brain that it's safe to lower cortisol and adrenaline output. Unlike intense exercise, which can ramp up alertness, gentle movement nudges your nervous system from "fight-or-flight" toward "rest-and-digest." Studies also show that mindful stretching or yoga sequences boost vagal tone, supporting the shift into recovery. The physical sensation of muscles lengthening and joints moving is itself a form of sensory reassurance that the crisis has passed.

A 5-Move Reset Routine You Can Do Anywhere

The right reset routine requires no equipment and little space. Below is a five-move sequence designed for after your shift, whether you're in a break room, at home, or alongside your car. Each movement should be performed slowly and consciously: focus on your breath, avoid pushing to extremes, and use the reset as active recovery, not a workout.

1. **Neck Release (30 seconds)**

   Sit or stand with your back straight. Drop your right ear toward your right shoulder and gently extend your left arm downward, feeling the stretch along the side of your neck. Hold for 15 seconds, then switch sides. This releases tension from hours of craning or bracing.

2. **Shoulder Roll and Stretch (1 minute)**

   Roll your shoulders up, back, and down in a circular motion 5–8 times. Then, interlace your fingers behind your back and gently straighten your arms, opening your chest. You'll notice immediate release through the upper back and chest, common hotspots for post-shift tension.

3. **Standing Forward Fold (1 minute)**

   Stand with feet hip-width apart. Allow your knees to soften as you hinge forward at the hips, letting your upper body drape toward the ground. Hold onto your elbows and gently sway left to right. This decompresses the spine and stretches your hamstrings after long hours standing or sitting.

4. **Seated Figure Four Stretch (1 minute)**

   Sit in a sturdy chair. Cross your right ankle over your left knee, flexing the right foot. Lean forward gently until you feel a stretch in your right hip and glute. Hold for 30 seconds, then repeat on the other side. This targets deep gluteal muscles that tighten up with long shifts or driving.

5. **Ankle Circles and Toe Flex (30 seconds each direction)**

   While seated or standing, lift one foot and slowly rotate your ankle through its full range in both directions. Then, flex and point your toes several times. Switch feet. This counters the foot and leg stiffness that can follow a demanding night on your feet.

Each move can be adapted: use a wall for balance, remain seated if needed, or pause briefly between stretches as your body allows.

Self-Check: Mobility and Tension Assessment

Knowing where you hold post-shift tension will make your movement routine more effective. Before your reset, quickly scan from head to toe and rate each key area using the scale below. This helps track patterns over time and gives instant feedback on your progress.

Printable Self-Rating Scale:

Rate each area 0–3 (0 = no tension/restriction, 3 = very tight/painful)

- ☐ Neck/Shoulders: 0 1 2 3
- ☐ Upper back/chest: 0 1 2 3
- ☐ Lower back: 0 1 2 3
- ☐ Hips/glutes: 0 1 2 3
- ☐ Feet/ankles: 0 1 2 3

You can print or jot down these ratings at the start and end of your reset. Look for any areas that consistently register high—this is where you might want to focus, modify, or add extra stretches.

Top Mistakes: Movements That Can Worsen Exhaustion or Disrupt Sleep

The goal isn't to break a sweat, it's to downshift. Certain habits, though common, can actually work against your reset:

- ***Performing high-intensity exercise post-shift (HIIT, running, vigorous cycling)***: These may spike adrenaline and make winding down harder.
- ***Static stretching held for too long or pushed to discomfort***: Overstretching can trigger soreness and micro-injury, making sleep uncomfortable.
- ***Ignoring pain or sharp discomfort***: Don't force through movements that cause real pain—stop and adapt as needed.
- ***Rapid, jerky movements***: Fast or ballistic movements activate rather than calm your nervous system.

If a stretch or movement feels stressful or brings on more fatigue, scale it back. The sequence should leave you feeling looser, calmer, and ready to wind down.

Modification Tips for Long Commutes and Minimal Time

A tight schedule or long drive doesn't mean you have to skip your reset. Here's how to adapt:

- ***Seated variations***: Most stretches above can be done in the driver's seat (car parked, engine off). Prioritize neck, shoulder, and ankle moves.
- ***Micro-doses***: If you only have two minutes, choose one or two areas that feel worst—say, shoulder rolls and ankle circles. Even one movement makes a difference.
- ***Break it up***: For commutes over 30 minutes, use a rest stop to do a standing forward fold or figure four stretch before resuming your drive.
- ***Schedule it***: Treat your micro-movement reset as part of your clock-out ritual. Even a short pause before getting out of the car or walking into your house solidifies the transition out of work mode.

In summary, adding structured, gentle movement to your after-shift toolkit primes your body for rest without overtaxing it. Micro-movements quickly help regulate nervous system arousal, release tension, and prepare you for better sleep. Reference the checklist and modify for your real-world constraints—you'll get more mileage out of every minute, no matter where you reset.

Chapter 6: Quick Environmental Tweaks to Signal 'Off Duty' to Your Brain

After gentle movement signals to your body that the shift is truly over, the next big lever is your physical environment. The cues you send your brain with light, sound, temperature, and even scent can either reinforce "on duty" alertness, or help nudge you toward real rest and recovery. Environmental tweaks aren't about elaborate renovations—they're small, targeted changes you can make before and after your shift to help your nervous system switch gears.

Step-by-step: Adjusting lights, noise, temperature for a post-shift wind-down

Start by focusing on lighting. Your brain's internal clock relies heavily on light cues. After a night shift, sunlight can be jarring and signal wakefulness just when you're aiming to wind down. On your way home, wear dark sunglasses, even if the sun isn't at full brightness yet. When you get inside, avoid overhead lights; use lamps with warm, dim bulbs instead. If you need to get ready for bed, try to keep the lighting as low as is safely possible.

Next, address sound. After a noisy clinical environment, your mind benefits from a predictable, gentle soundscape. White noise machines work well, since they block out sudden noises that might otherwise jar you awake as you try to sleep. If you don't have a machine, a steady fan or an audio app set on rainfall or ambient hum can serve the same purpose.

Temperature plays a larger role than many realize. Your core body temperature needs to drop slightly for restful sleep. Aim for a room that feels a few degrees cooler than your work environment, ideally between 60-67°F (16-19°C). If you share your space, consider a fan directed at your side of the bed, or a cooling mattress pad for more control.

Deliverable: Checklist for prepping your sleep space before your shift begins Forward-thinking pays dividends for shift workers. Before your next shift starts, set up your sleep haven so you can unwind as soon as you walk in the door. Use this quick checklist:

- Blackout window coverings drawn fully (or blackout shades ready to pull down)
- White noise machine, fan, or trusted app set up and ready to switch on
- Warm, dim lighting options by your bed (avoid turning on main room lights after shift)
- Bed linens fresh and inviting, with your preferred pillow easily accessible
- Room cooled to your preferred sleep temperature (set thermostat or fan timer)

- Sleep mask and earplugs in reach, just in case outside factors are unavoidable
- Any calming scent (lavender spray, roll-on essential oil, sachet) placed by the bed

Doing these small steps ahead of time means you bypass friction, and reduce the willpower needed to follow through while tired.

Home vs. car: Adapting your environment on the go

Your wind-down doesn't have to wait until you're in bed. Many clinicians decompress in the car or during a commute. If you arrive home and others are awake, or if you nap before driving, small tweaks help wherever you are:

- Window shades or sun visors in your car block incoming light if you need a rest before driving.
- Stash foam earplugs in your work bag, glove compartment, or jacket pocket for instant noise reduction—even on public transit.
- Keep a calming scent in the car, lavender, cedar, or another non-stimulating aroma. A vent clip or a small cotton ball with essential oil works without overpowering.

If your commute is long, try playing soft instrumental music or soothing podcasts, not alerting, energetic content.

Making these changes portable ensures your transition cues are always within reach, even if your routine gets disrupted.

Avoiding "wakeful triggers": Identifying and eliminating stimuli that delay reset

Some environmental factors actively fight against your ability to shut down after a shift. Identifying these triggers—and removing or reducing them—helps avoid that frustrating "tired but wired" state.

The biggest culprits are bright, blue-tinged lights (like phone and tablet screens), household noise (loud voices, TVs, kitchen activity), and unfamiliar or sharp smells (cooking odors, strong cleaners). To minimize wakeful triggers:

- Set up your phone for "night mode" or use a blue light filter app before heading home.
- Ask housemates or family to keep TVs and voices down during your intended sleep window.
- Time household chores or meal prep for later in the day, or close your door if strong smells reach your room.

Be methodical. Walk through your home once during daylight and once when preparing for sleep, noting anything you find alerting. Take small steps to buffer or block those triggers.

Troubleshooting: Small-space/ roommate/household-specific modifications for clinicians

Not everyone has a private, quiet suite to sleep in. Many clinicians share space or live in busy households. Still, practical modifications can stack the deck in your favor.

For small or shared rooms:

- Invest in a quality sleep mask and multi-use earplugs for consistent darkness and quiet.
- Use room dividers or portable screens to carve out a visual barrier and define your rest area.
- Keep a basket by your bed with sleep essentials (mask, earplugs, calming spray) so they're always on hand.

If you have roommates or family:

- Establish clear, written (or texted) quiet hours. A sticky note or signal outside your door communicates your sleep time without repeated explanations.
- Use a white noise app on your phone if a physical machine isn't feasible.
- Consider hanging a towel or heavy fabric over your door and windows as a makeshift sound and light buffer.

In tight, multi-use spaces:

- Try a cot or sleeping pad you can set up when off-duty and stash away later.

- Store a small, foldable fan under your bed for portable cooling and white noise.

Every home is different, and not every fix works for every living arrangement. Instead, prioritize what you can control: sensory input (light, noise, scent), and setting up your sleep space for the fewest surprises possible.

Wrapping up, quick environmental tweaks are rarely glamorous, but their impact can be profound. Clinicians who master these cues find themselves falling asleep faster, resting deeper, and recovering more completely—regardless of living situation or external noise. When you build these steps into your routine, you create a powerful signal: the shift has ended, and it's truly time to go off duty.

Chapter 7: Mastering the Transition Ritual—Shifting from Work to Recovery Mode

Mastering the shift from a high-alert, professional mindset to genuine recovery is not something that happens on its own. Even after tweaking your physical environment to support winding down, there remains a crucial, often overlooked step: the transition ritual. For clinicians and EMS professionals, an intentional ritual acts as a psychological "off switch," signaling your brain and body that the demands of the shift are over. Get this right, and you pave the way for real rest. Rush or neglect it, and stress lingers far past the end of your shift.

Why ritual matters: Psychological transitions from crisis mode to personal mode

When work is defined by unpredictability and urgency, your nervous system rarely settles the moment you clock out. Emergency response, critical care, or even routine night rounds require a level of vigilance that has to be purposefully wound down. Without a formal transition ritual, you carry "crisis mode" home with you, whether that shows up as racing thoughts, physical tension, or feeling detached from your personal life.

A well-crafted ritual tunes your nervous system for recovery. It tells your brain, "the critical phase is done; safe mode begins now." This psychological boundary isn't just nice to have, it's a functional tool that reduces intrusive replay, lowers physiological arousal, and primes your mind for personal connection, rest, or sleep. Anchor this transition with simple, repeatable actions, and your body will start to recognize and respond to those cues, automatically easing off the gas.

Three sample rituals to shift gears

If you're new to intentional transition rituals, start simple. Here are three field-tested rituals especially suited for night-shifters:

"Uniform off" process: Instead of simply changing out of your workwear, turn this act into a signal to your nervous system. For some, this is as structured as removing each item with mindful intent—naming, in your mind or out loud, what you're leaving behind (e.g., "Jacket off; I'm no longer on call"). Place your uniform or gear in its designated spot rather than leaving it in a heap. This small ceremony marks a clear end to your shift identity.

Gratitude logging: Keep a small notebook or digital list in your bag or at your bedside. After your shift, write down one or two things that went well, or one person or moment you appreciated. This short practice doesn't deny the tough parts of your shift, but it reorients your mind toward balance. Gratitude practice has been shown to lower stress and improve mental recovery, making it a solid addition to your transition toolkit.

Quick digital detox: Set your phone to Do Not Disturb or enable a “wind-down” mode as soon as your shift ends. Use the first 10–15 minutes after work to avoid social media, emails, and news. Instead, engage in a brief analog activity, stretching, gentle movement, or simply deep breathing. By temporarily detaching from digital noise, you allow your nervous system to reset without additional demands.

Template: Script your own reset ritual with cues and rewards

Your transition ritual should match your habits, work environment, and stress triggers.

Consider this framework for designing your personalized ritual:

1. ***Pick a cue***: Anchor the ritual to an existing event. This could be stepping through your front door, sitting in your car post-shift, or even the act of removing your badge.
2. ***Choose 1–2 actions***: These are deliberate, repeatable steps. Options include:
    - ☐ Changing clothes with intention.

- ☐ Washing your hands and face with slow, focused attention.
- ☐ Logging gratitude or lessons learned (a single sentence will do).
- ☐ Putting away your work equipment methodically.
- ☐ Practicing two minutes of slow breathing, eyes closed.

3. ***Identify a reward***: Give yourself a small, satisfying reward at the end. This isn't about indulgence; it's a signal your brain can associate with "work is over." A hot shower, your favorite snack, or settling into bed with a book all work. The reward needs to be immediate and consistent—to reinforce the ritual.
4. ***Stick to a sequence***: Repeating the steps, in order, helps them become automatic over time.
5. ***To script your own ritual***: Write down your cue, 1–2 core actions, and your chosen reward.

Keep this plan somewhere visible. Practice the ritual for a week, then adjust as needed.

Metrics: How to track your transition ritual's success

Measuring a transition ritual isn't about perfection—it's about noticing if it serves its purpose. Use these straightforward methods to keep tabs on your progress:

- ☐ ***Self-check***: After your ritual, rate your tension, irritability, or "mental stuckness" on a simple scale (e.g., 0–10). Do this before and after, if you have a moment.
- ☐ ***Sleep onset***: Notice if you're able to fall asleep more easily after the ritual. Track your average time to sleep or note the number of nights you toss and turn.
- ☐ ***Intrusive thoughts***: Pay attention to the frequency of work-related thoughts once you're home. If these decrease after your ritual, you're making headway.
- ☐ ***Partner or housemate feedback***: Ask those you live with if they notice any difference in your presence, mood, or responsiveness after your routine.

Choose one or two indicators and track your results for at least a week before making changes. Sometimes just the act of checking in heightens your awareness and commitment.

Common errors—rituals that backfire or reinforce stress

Not all rituals help. Some actually keep you stuck in "on duty" mode or even amplify stress.

Watch for these common pitfalls:

- ***Overcomplication***: If your ritual has too many steps or is hard to remember, it increases pressure rather than decreases it. Simplicity is key.

- ***Unintentional rumination***: If your ritual always involves replaying difficult cases or venting about work, you risk deepening stress. The reset should create distance, not reinforce the work mindset.
- ***Digital drift***: "Checking out" by scrolling through emails or social media often prolongs nervous system activation and delays true recovery.
- ***Neglecting physical cues***: Skipping the tangible elements (changing clothes, washing up, turning off badge tones) leaves your brain anchored to the work state.
- ***Inconsistency***: If the ritual is applied only sporadically, the signal weakens. Routine builds power through repetition.

Effective transition rituals anchor you in the present, give your mind and body a reliable "shift end" signal, and pave the way for quality rest and recovery. Choose your approach consciously, keep it simple, and review your results regularly. The right ritual becomes less an obligation and more a trusted ally as you master the art of transitioning from duty to downtime.

Chapter 8: Caffeine and Nutrition for the Night-Shift Clinician

As you step out of the post-shift ritual and begin your wind-down, what you consume, caffeine, meals, or snacks, can either set you up for efficient recovery or quietly undermine your ability to rest. Night-shift clinicians know the hazards of sleep deprivation, but it's easy to underestimate the role that caffeine timing and nutrition play in supporting your nervous system. Fine-tuning these areas can help you transition from high-alert work mode to real, restorative downtime.

Caffeine Metabolism After the Shift

Caffeine is a mainstay for many clinicians working overnight. However, its stimulating effects linger far longer than most expect. After ingestion, caffeine peaks in the bloodstream within 30–60 minutes, but its half-life ranges from about 5 to 7 hours, depending on your genetics, age, and overall health. That means if you swallow your last cup of strong coffee at 4 a.m., you may still have substantial caffeine circulating at noon when you're trying to sleep.

Residual caffeine doesn't just keep you awake; it also lowers sleep quality by fragmenting deep and REM sleep, which are crucial for physical and mental reset. This is why even "feeling sleepy" after a shift can be misleading, your body may be fatigued, but your nervous system is still partially activated, blocking genuine restorative rest.

Checklist: Best and Worst Foods for After-Shift Recovery

What you eat following a night on duty can ease your transition into sleep or drive further alertness and agitation. Here's a quick-reference guide for food choices post-shift:

Best Foods for Recovery:

- ***Complex carbohydrates*** (whole grains, oats, brown rice): Support serotonin production, allowing a natural wind-down.
- ***Lean proteins*** (turkey, chicken, tofu, eggs): Help stabilize blood sugar and provide amino acids for tissue repair.
- ***Magnesium-rich foods*** (spinach, pumpkin seeds, almonds): Promote muscle relaxation and nervous system calming.
- ***Fermented foods*** (yogurt, kefir, kimchi): Benefit gut health, which impacts mood regulation and overall stress response.
- ***Hydrating fruits and vegetables*** (cucumber, watermelon, berries): Rehydrate and deliver micronutrients lost during the shift.

Foods to Avoid After Your Shift:

- ***High-sugar items*** (pastries, candy, sugar-laden cereals): Cause energy spikes and crashes, disrupting the ability to wind down.
- ***Heavy/fried foods*** (fast food burgers, fries): Slow digestion and contribute to gastrointestinal discomfort during sleep.
- ***Large, high-protein meals*** (steaks, protein bars): Take longer to digest, potentially leading to restless or fragmented sleep.
- ***Excessive sodium*** (take-out, canned soups): Promotes dehydration and may increase nighttime blood pressure.
- ***Spicy foods***: May trigger heartburn or raise core body temperature, making it harder to fall asleep.

Timing Your Last Caffeine Intake

To optimize recovery, you need to intentionally time your caffeine "cut-off." The right window will depend on your shift's end time and how quickly you hope to transition to sleep after clocking out.

Use this decision tool to find your best fit:

- ☐ Determine your shift end time and typical bedtime (when you actually aim to sleep, not just when you get home).

- ☐ Count back at least 6 hours from that sleep time. This is your ideal latest point for consuming caffeine.
- ☐ Example: Shift ends at 7 a.m., home by 8 a.m., sleep goal by 9 a.m.—latest caffeine should be no later than 3 a.m.
- ☐ If your sleep latency (how quickly you fall asleep) is consistently under 15 minutes, you may be able to experiment with a cut-off as little as 4–5 hours pre-bed.
- ☐ If you experience racing thoughts, fitful sleep, or repeated wake-ups, push your caffeine cut-off even earlier and consider switching to decaf or non-caffeinated drinks in the final hours of your shift.

  Remember, energy drinks, sodas, iced teas, and certain medications also contain caffeine.

- ☐ Read labels closely during the post-midnight stretch.

Sample 24-Hour Recovery Meal Plan

Here's a framework for structuring nutrition on a recovery day following a night shift, aiming for stable energy and smoother wind-down:

Post-Shift (within 30–60 minutes after clock-out):

- ***Hydration***: 1–2 glasses of water, possibly with a splash of electrolyte solution.

- ***Light meal/snack***: Whole-grain toast with nut butter and sliced banana, or overnight oats with berries and seeds.

Pre-Sleep (about 30 minutes before bed):

Small, sleep-supportive snack: Greek yogurt with a sprinkle of granola, or a small bowl of unsweetened cereal with milk. Avoid caffeine, chocolate, or anything overly heavy.

Upon Waking (after main daytime sleep period):

- ***Hydrating refresh***: Water or herbal tea.
- ***Balanced meal***: Quinoa or brown rice bowl with grilled chicken or tofu, leafy greens, roasted vegetables, and a small fruit serving.

Mid-"Day" (afternoon/evening, before next shift):

- ***Protein and carbs***: Turkey and vegetable wrap, lentil soup, or a sweet potato with cottage cheese and avocado.
- ***Snacks as needed***: Raw nuts, cut veggies with hummus, or a small fruit smoothie.

Before Next Shift:

- ***Final meal before work***: Moderate portion, not overly heavy—think brown rice, steamed fish, sautéed greens.

  The key here is moderation—meals should support sleep, not induce sluggishness or spikes.

- Adjust to your appetite and personal digestive comfort.

Nutritional Pitfalls: Late-Night Eating That Sabotages Recovery

Late-night eating sometimes feels unavoidable after a physically and emotionally draining shift. But certain habits can work against your reset goals:

- Consuming large, greasy, or spicy meals close to bedtime can trigger indigestion, acid reflux, and elevated core temperature, all of which prolong sleep onset.
- Near-binge eating or grazing on high-sugar foods can cause a fast drop in blood sugar later, which may wake you up mid-sleep or worsen grogginess upon waking.
- Excess use of caffeine-containing snacks or “energy bars” marketed for recovery can unknowingly delay sleep drive.

To counter these pitfalls:

- Plan your after-shift snack before leaving work, so you aren’t left rooting for junk food in exhaustion.
- Favor single servings of whole foods rather than mindlessly snacking.
- Practice a brief mindfulness check before eating: Are you hungry, thirsty, or simply exhausted? This helps prevent emotionally-driven overeating.

Wrapping Up

Caffeine and nutrition are foundational, but often neglected players in the night-shift recovery process. Thoughtful timing of your last caffeine dose, careful selection of recovery foods, and structure around post-shift meals do more than fuel your body; they actively prepare your nervous system for quality sleep. By refining what and when you eat and drink after a shift, you take another concrete step toward sustainable, healthy night-shift work.

Chapter 9: Sleep Hygiene—Evidence-Based Habits for Deep, Restful Daytime Sleep

Building sustainable restful sleep after a night shift is an uphill battle for most clinicians and EMS staff. Your biology is fighting daylight, family demands, and the ingrained routines of a world designed for daytime living. Fortunately, research-backed sleep hygiene practices can tip the odds in your favor. This chapter condenses those findings into an actionable, real-world system that fits your unpredictable life and household.

Comprehensive Checklist: Your Daytime Sleep Fundamentals

Creating a reliable sleep environment is foundational. Below is a focused checklist for immediate, proven impact:

- ☐ Limit light exposure in the hour before bed. Shield your eyes with sunglasses on the way home, and avoid device screens or install blue light filters.
- ☐ Invest in blackout curtains. Make your bedroom truly dark, no stray light from windows or electronics.
- ☐ Use a white noise machine or a fan. This helps mask abrupt household or street sounds that disrupt light sleep.

- ☐ Consider earplugs if outside or household noise is consistent. There are comfortable, low-profile options suitable for side sleepers.
- ☐ Maintain a cool room temperature. Aim for 60–67°F (16–19°C) if possible; overheating fragments REM and deep sleep.
- ☐ Experiment with sleep-promoting scents. Lavender, chamomile, or cedar oil in a diffuser can support relaxation, but keep it subtle and avoid overpowering fragrances.
- ☐ Block morning daylight exposure during your commute. Use wraparound sunglasses and a hat to prevent your brain from "morning mode" activation.
- ☐ Turn your phone to "Do Not Disturb," silencing notifications, alarms, or vibration.
- ☐ Avoid caffeine in the last 6–8 hours before bed, as outlined in the previous chapter.

Step-by-Step: Layering Evidence-Based Sleep Habits

High-yield sleep routines are most effective when stacked in a deliberate order. Here's how to layer these habits for maximum effect, even if you're exhausted and short on time:

- Wind down at work or during your commute with a calming ritual, breathing, music, or a brief mindfulness practice.

- Slip into “sleep mode” as soon as you enter your bedroom. Close blackout curtains fully, power off lights and screens, and set up your noise machine or fan right away.
- Choose comfortable sleepwear and bedding dedicated only for sleep (avoid using the same clothes you wore during your shift).
- If you struggle to fall asleep, use aromatherapy or a warm (not hot) shower to help transition your mind and body.
- Keep hydration modest. Drink enough water post-shift to rehydrate, but avoid large amounts that could wake you overnight to use the bathroom.
- Repeat a brief, calming ritual (gentle stretching, gratitude thoughts, or slow breathing) as your final step before bed.

Don’t try changing everything simultaneously. Target one or two habits at a time, then build as you notice improvement.

Examples: Using a Sleep Diary to Track Progress

Tracking sleep habits helps cut through guesswork and reveals patterns you might miss. A simple sleep diary template can clarify which interventions actually help. Use the following sample fields:

- ***Date:***
- ***Time into bed:***

- ***Estimated time to fall asleep:***
- ***Number of times woken:***
- ***Time out of bed:***
- ***Sleep interruptions (noise, light, temperature, thoughts):***
- ***Habits before bed (wind-down, caffeine, screens, etc.):***
- ***Sleep quality (1–5 scale):***

Keep your entries brief. For a digital version, consider free apps designed for shift workers, but don't get bogged down by elaborate features—a simple notes app or paper log works fine. Review a week at a time to spot which changes give you the best return.

Troubleshooting: When Sleep is Fragmented or Elusive

Even with good habits, daytime sleep is prone to interruptions. Here's how to troubleshoot the most common problems:

- ***Waking frequently***: Confirm that your sleep space is truly dark and quiet. Even brief exposure to sunlight or noise can trigger wakefulness. If family or roommate noise is a factor, post a sign or agree on quiet hours during your sleep window.
- ***Trouble falling asleep***: Re-check caffeine intake, and avoid heavy or spicy meals before bed. If racing

thoughts persist, use a timed worry-journal session or repeat calming breathwork.

- ***Light sleep or unrefreshing rest***: Lower the room temperature and consider rotating bedding for comfort. Experiment with a weighted blanket, but discontinue if it increases restlessness.
- ***Extremely short sleep duration***: If your window for sleep is tight, focus on maximizing sleep efficiency with darker rooms, noise protection, and by aligning naps strategically before or after main sleep.

If after significant efforts you regularly get less than 4–5 hours of sleep, consider consulting a sleep specialist for further evaluation.

Home and Family Adaptation: Building a Sleep-Support Culture

Daytime sleep is not just a personal issue—it's a household or family one. For clinicians sharing space with partners, children, or roommates, some adaptation is necessary to make deep sleep possible:

- Communicate clearly about your sleep hours. Post a visible schedule on the door or fridge so others know when you are "out of service."
- Problem-solve with housemates about routine sources of noise or disruption (e.g., vacuuming, dog walking, loud calls).

- Use batch meal prep or order groceries online to cut down on household tasks close to your sleep time.
- For families, coordinate quiet activities during your sleep window—screen time with headphones, homework hour, or silent reading period.
- If space allows, designate a separate sleep area from shared family living zones.
- Express appreciation for household support—small thanks reinforce cooperation and help sustain routines.

Remind yourself and others that quality sleep after night shift is not a luxury, but a necessity for safety and health. Buy-in from those around you can be the difference between cumulative sleep loss and sustainable recovery.

Wrapping Up

Building better sleep as a night-shift clinician is an ongoing project, not a one-time overhaul. Every environment and household is unique, but layering simple, proven habits, controlling light, sound, temperature, and routine, makes a real, immediate difference. Use the checklist above to prioritize, track your progress with a diary, and adapt your approach as you go. If setbacks occur, troubleshoot directly or reset expectations with those you live with. With evidence-based strategies and consistent adaptation, deep, restorative sleep can become a reliable part of your recovery, even when the world is just waking up.

Chapter 10: Calming Tools for Persistent Hyperarousal

Even when you optimize your sleep environment, many clinicians and EMS professionals still battle stubborn hyperarousal after night shifts. Restlessness, rapid heart rate, and a sense of being on high alert can linger long past the end of your shift. This chapter zeroes in on practical calming tools you can deploy when basic wind-downs are not enough.

Quick Wins: Simple Tools with Immediate Calming Impact

Certain physical and sensory tools can quickly dial down a ramped-up nervous system. Four standouts—acupressure mats, weighted blankets, guided audio, and blue blocker glasses—offer rapid relief when persistently keyed up. Here's how they work:

- Acupressure mats use short, firm plastic spikes that stimulate pressure points. Lying back for five to ten minutes can prompt a gentle endorphin release and activate the body's relaxation response. Most people feel a noticeable drop in muscle tension and mind chatter within the first session.
- Weighted blankets provide gentle, evenly distributed pressure. This "deep touch" sensation has been shown to lower heart rate and decrease physiological arousal,

making it easier to transition toward sleep even when your mind is spinning.

- Guided audio, such as progressive relaxation tracks, soundscapes, or sleep-specific meditations, shifts your focus away from internal stress. Audio tools create enough sensory distraction to drown out intrusive thoughts or "mental replay" after tough shifts.
- Blue blocker glasses filter out stimulating blue-spectrum light from screens and indoor lighting. Wearing these glasses on the commute home or during any wind-down prep helps cue your body that it's time to shut down, supporting melatonin production and reducing overstimulation.

Layering Physical and Sensory Tools for Maximum Effect

You'll often get the fastest relief when you combine—or "layer"—calming tools. Think of this as assembling a custom toolkit: using two or three interventions simultaneously can nudge your system from hyperarousal into a state where sleep is finally possible.

To layer these tools effectively:

1. Start physical, then add sensory inputs. Lie down on an acupressure mat for five minutes while listening to a calming audio track. Focus on steady nasal breathing.

2. After rising from the mat, slip under a weighted blanket. Keep your blue blocker glasses on if light exposure is still an issue.
3. If you're in a brightly lit home, switch overheads to dim, warm-toned bulbs or continue using blue blocker glasses until you're ready to close your eyes.

Experiment with timing. Some find that a short stint with each tool (five to ten minutes) back to back is ideal. Others benefit more from overlapping—such as using a weighted blanket while an audio meditation plays.

Matching Calming Tools to Your Own Stress Patterns

Not all stress after a shift feels the same, so personalization pays off. Use the following short worksheet (you can jot this in a notebook or notes app) to match tools to your patterns:

Identify Your Stress State:

- Acute anxiety (racing heart, shallow breathing, restless energy)
- Chronic tension (tight shoulders, jaw clenching, persistent irritability) Wired but tired (mentally exhausted, body restless, trouble "switching off")

Pinpoint Your Triggers:

Is it replaying events from the shift? Anticipating family responsibilities? Overstimulation from lights/screens? Use honest, specific language.

Try, Then Match Tools:

- ***For acute anxiety***: Start with the weighted blanket and add guided audio.
- ***For chronic body tension***: Begin with the acupressure mat, then layer dim lighting with blue blocker glasses.
- ***For mental hyperactivity***: Prioritize guided meditation or sleep stories with sensory dampening (eye mask, dim room).

Record What Works:

After each attempt, make a simple note: Did this combo help you feel calmer? Did you fall asleep faster? Adjust based on results.

Rapid Guide: Which Calming Tool to Use, When

Knowing which tool is best at the moment can save precious time when you're depleted.

- ***Acute anxiety*** (unsettling panic, physical unease): Reach for the weighted blanket first—this grounds your body fast. Pair it with a progressive muscle relaxation audio if thoughts are spiraling.

- ***Chronic baseline stress*** (ongoing tension but functional): Use blue blocker glasses as soon as your shift ends, then incorporate an acupressure mat to release accumulated physical stress.
- ***"Tired but wired" or mental replay***: Guided sleep meditations and sensory reduction (dim lighting, eye masks) work best. Skip highly stimulating inputs—even minor device usage can derail your effort.

If you're unsure, stack two different tools and note which helps most. This process is about practical trial-and-error, not perfection.

Pitfalls: Calming Tools That Can Backfire

Even effective tools have limitations—not every option suits every person or every night. Be mindful of these common pitfalls, especially for clinicians used to powering through discomfort.

Weighted blankets aren't for everyone. If you have respiratory concerns, chronic pain, or a strong aversion to confined sensations, using one may be counterproductive. Test with a lighter or smaller blanket first if you're uncertain.

Acupressure mats can overstimulate sensitive or anxious individuals—if your discomfort rises after a minute or two, swap out for a less intense tool, such as a simple foam roller or gentle yoga stretch.

Guided audio can backfire if the content features unexpected sounds (e.g., bird calls, heavy rain, or sudden voices) that activate your alert system. Choose short playlists you've previewed. Avoid new audios when you're deeply overtired.

Blue blocker glasses only work if they actually filter the correct spectrum—and some people will find wearing glasses at all adds extra irritability. If you notice headaches or eye strain, prioritize turning down screens instead.

Finally, avoid "stacking" so many new tools at once that the effort itself becomes overwhelming. Start with one or two interventions you're curious about and build gradually.

Consistency wins out over novelty.

Wrapping Up and Looking Ahead

Persistent hyperarousal can feel inescapable, but the right set of sensory and physical tools can help restore a sense of control—even when your environment and schedule work against you. Use the tools and worksheet here to refine your own after-shift reset, adjusting combinations as your stress patterns evolve. The next chapter will tackle strategies for managing the intrusive thoughts and mental replays that often follow a tough shift, building on the foundation you've set for calming your body and nervous system.

Chapter 11: Managing Intrusive Thoughts and Mental Replay

For night-shift clinicians and EMS workers, intrusive thoughts and replaying the shift's events can sabotage even the best sleep routines. The mind tends to rehash patient encounters, decisions under pressure, or moments where the outcome was less than ideal. This chapter provides real, actionable tools to help you put the workday to rest—mentally as well as physically.

Setting a Psychological "Shift End" With Writing or Recording

One of the most effective ways to close the mental door on your shift is by establishing a psychological cutoff. This isn't about ignoring what happened or pretending stress doesn't exist. Instead, you're creating a clear mental signpost that your responsibility for the shift has ended.

Take two to five minutes at the end of each shift—even if you're exhausted—to jot down or record on your phone a brief summary of three key points:

- One thing that went well (no matter how small).
- One thing that was difficult or unsolved.
- One acknowledgement: Tell yourself, "My shift is over. I have done what I can for today." You can use a

dedicated notebook, a secure app, or your phone's voice recorder. The point is not a perfect account; it's to signal to your brain that you have registered your thoughts and can lay them down for now. For many, this ritual acts like punching out of work before heading home, helping reduce the tendency for mental replay later.

Decision Checklist: Choosing Your Response Tool

Intrusive thoughts vary—some are flashes of worry, some are loops of regret or what-ifs. Not all response tools work for every kind. Instead of defaulting to rumination or avoidance, use this quick checklist to decide which approach might serve you best:

Use thought-stopping techniques if:

- ☐ You catch yourself replaying the same scene repeatedly with no new insight.
- ☐ The thought interrupts your attempts to relax, sleep, or engage in recovery.

Try guided imagery if:

- ☐ Your mind is stuck on emotionally loaded memories or unresolved stress.
- ☐ Relaxation feels physically impossible because of lingering adrenaline.

Shift to cognitive refocus if:

- You notice yourself "filling in the blanks" with negative predictions ("I know I missed something—what if it goes wrong?").
- You feel trapped in fault-finding or spiraling hypothetical scenarios.

In practice, this means recognizing when the thought reel starts, pausing, and actively choosing a response strategy. Not every tool will yield immediate relief every time; consistency is what helps retrain mental patterns over time.

5-Minute "Mental Containment" Process: Step-by-Step

When intrusive replay threatens to overwhelm, use this structured containment exercise. It's not about ignoring reality but about containing its impact until you are rested enough to process it properly.

- Sit in a quiet space and set a timer for five minutes.
- Bring to mind the most persistent thought or scene from your shift.
- Picture that thought as a physical object—a file, a room, a box.
- Name the emotion attached to it (stress, guilt, irritation).

- Visualize placing the thought-object into a container (a locked drawer, a box with a lid). Tell yourself: "This is here if I need it—but I choose to set it aside until later. I am off duty." Take three slow breaths focusing on what you want to do next (sleep, eat, decompress).

You can combine visual cues—like shutting a notebook or turning off an audio note—to reinforce the exercise. Repetition teaches your mind to accept boundaries between work stress and personal recovery.

Night Shift Rumination Traps: What to Watch For

Night-shift settings create specific traps for mental replay, often more stubborn than those faced by daytime colleagues. Some common pitfalls include:

- ***Replay amplified by isolation***: With fewer social outlets post-shift, you may find yourself ruminating because there's no conversational outlet to process the day.
- ***"Hero trap" thinking***: A sense that you alone are responsible for every outcome can make letting go especially hard. This trap often fuels late-night anxiety and insomnia.
- ***Problem-solving at the wrong time***: Your brain tries to "finish the work" off the clock. You might feel

compelled to double-check protocols or message colleagues after hours, keeping your mind on duty.

Recognizing these patterns is the first step to defusing them. Set clear digital and mental boundaries (no checking charts, no scrolling patient files) after your mental containment exercise.

Self-Assessment: Tracking Frequency and Intensity

Monitoring intrusive thoughts gives you objective feedback and can highlight when patterns worsen or improve. Simple tracking will also help you identify which tools and rituals are working.

Try a nightly, rapid check-in, either written or on your phone, with these questions:

- *How many times tonight have I caught myself replaying shift events?*
- *How strong is the urge to return to these thoughts (mild, moderate, intense)?*
- *Which tool did I use (writing, guided imagery, containment, etc.)?*
- *Did it reduce the mental "charge" or not?*

This isn't meant to become another task to worry over. Keep it brief and factual; if you notice rising intensity or frequency over days or weeks, this is a clear signal to tweak your reset strategies or consider reaching out to a support resource.

Bringing It Together

Intrusive thoughts do not mean you're failing at recovery. They're a predictable response to demanding, high-stakes work. But left unchecked, chronic mental replay of the night shift undermines rest, mood, and readiness for the next cycle.

By establishing a psychological "shift end," using a targeted intervention, and tracking your patterns with discipline, you gain back control over your off-duty hours. Practicing these tools isn't about eliminating your sense of responsibility. It's about protecting your ability to recover and sustain your vital work. The next chapter will show how brief, intentional connection with others can further reinforce your post-shift reset and help close the loop on a demanding night.

Chapter 12: The Power of Micro-Connection: Social Recovery After the Shift

The end of a night shift doesn't always mean you're ready to reconnect. The exhaustion, hyperarousal, or mental replay you experience can leave you craving silence and solitude.

But cutting off entirely from others, even for what feels like recovery, carries real risks. Micro-connection, the art of brief and intentional social moments, offers a valuable alternative. Rather than a draining conversation or forced engagement, it's about small check-ins that help ground you and support mental health, without sapping the last of your energy.

Significance of Brief, Intentional Connection (and Its Opposite)

Social withdrawal can feel like the only plausible answer post-shift, especially after intense or traumatic calls. It's understandable to seek quiet. But entirely disconnecting for days or falling into prolonged isolation can amplify fatigue, worsen low mood, and erode your sense of belonging, key factors in night-shift burnout. Even short, sincere contact does more than just update others; it maintains social "anchors" that promote psychological stability.

Micro-connection doesn't mean deep conversation or social outings. It might be a quick text to a partner, a 60-second call, or a single voice note to a close friend. These small gestures signal, both to you and your support system, that you're still part of a network. Brief connection interrupts the feedback loop of isolation, offering moments of validation or even just acknowledgment.

Action Plan: 3-Minute Communication Templates

To make these connections practical, create a set of go-to templates that let you check in without overcommitting. The idea is to use just a few minutes, making the barrier as low as possible. If words or energy feel hard to summon, a template keeps you from getting stuck.

Try these options for check-ins, each designed to be sent or recorded in under three minutes:

Text template to family:

"Off my shift and heading home. Feeling wiped, but wanted to let you know I'm okay. Need to decompress—will check in after I rest. Hope your morning's going smoothly."

Text template to a peer/partner:

"That was a tough shift, but I made it through. Just checking in—hope things are alright on your end. I'll catch up more later once I've recharged."

Voice note template example:

"Hey, just wanted to say I'm done for the night. I might be slow to reply but wanted to touch base. Hope you're good—will reach out soon when I'm less foggy."

The key is clarity and brevity. Don't feel obligated to explain everything or be fully present. The main message: you're safe, you acknowledge the other person, and you have a plan to reconnect later if needed.

Checklist: Solitude or Support?

Some days, connection feels possible. Other days, you might need true silence. Recognizing what you need requires honesty—both for your sake and so others don't misinterpret distancing. Use this quick self-check before defaulting to withdrawal:

- ☐ Do I feel resentful or anxious at the thought of any contact right now?
- ☐ Am I truly recharging through solitude, or am I avoiding interaction out of numbness or overwhelm?

- ☐ Have I gone two or more consecutive days without meaningful contact outside of work?
- ☐ Do I need to say "I'm off-limits" or do I need someone to notice I'm struggling?

If your answers lean toward needing support (especially if isolation is extending beyond a day or two), shift toward a micro-connection with someone you trust. If you clearly need solitude, communicate it: "I need some quiet time right after shift—will text later." Cue others with a clear timeline.

How to Cue for Your Needs

If you live with family or share space, nonverbal signals can prime your household. For example, headphones on or a post-it ("Resting—back in 2 hours") can gently set boundaries without awkwardness. Consider building routines, like a fixed "check-in time" after sleep, so your absence isn't seen as withdrawal. If you prefer minimal communication, one emoji or "decompressing, will check in by _____" sets expectations.

Examples: Rapid Check-in Templates

Much of the friction around social recovery is the worry of "not doing enough" or seeming cold. Rapid check-ins, done right, replace apologies with matter-of-fact updates. Here are samples you can adapt:

- Quick text to a friend:

"Home safe, totally drained, but sending a quick hey so you know I'm okay."

- Short reply to group chat:

  "Alive but exhausted, catch you all tomorrow!"

- Audio note:

  "Off shift, shutting down for now. Thanks for checking in, talk soon when I'm upright."

Remember, the purpose isn't a conversation. It's simply to put a marker out there: "I'm here, I'll be back, but I'm recovering." Use whichever format feels least taxing, or create shortcuts on your phone for recurring messages.

Warning Signs: When Isolation Becomes Risk

Most night-shift clinicians report waves of wanting to disappear for a while. Occasional withdrawal is healthy. Persistent isolation is not. Watch for the following cues that it's time to seek more active connection:

- More than two days without any non-work contact.
- Increasing irritability or feeling "shut down" around loved ones, even after rest.
- Dread or anxiety at the thought of reconnecting with anyone, even close friends.

- Notifying contacts less and less, to the point of "ghosting."
- Noticing that sleep, mood, or appetite are worsening in tandem with isolation.

If you recognize these patterns, take one small step: send a micro-check-in rather than waiting to "feel better" first. Early action prevents small social gaps from widening into chronic loneliness or burnout.

Closing Perspective

Post-shift recovery is more than just physical rest or sleep hygiene.

Micro-connection—brief, thoughtful moments of social contact—can be a stabilizer through relentless cycles of exhaustion. You don't have to be the life of the party or even say much. Just show up, for a moment, in someone else's world. And when you truly need a break, communicate it openly. This balance of solitude and connection isn't just protective; over time, it helps preserve the sense of community that sustains you in a demanding role.

In the next chapter, you'll see how to use strategic napping and re-entry routines to go from exhausted to functional as you transition deeper into recovery.

Chapter 13: Strategic Napping and Re-Entry Routines

Transitioning out of night mode isn't always as simple as socializing or winding down. Sometimes, exhaustion or wired alertness calls for a targeted reset, one that helps bridge the gap between the end of your shift and quality sleep. Strategic napping and effective re-entry routines can play a crucial role in making that transition smoother, sharper, and safer for busy clinicians and EMS workers.

Evidence on nap timing, duration, and sleep inertia control for shift workers

Unlike full sleep episodes, strategic naps are precise tools. A well-timed nap has been shown to counter acute sleep debt, reduce error rates, and even support mood after a punishing shift. Research across shift-working professions consistently highlights three key factors: timing, duration, and management of sleep inertia (that groggy, disoriented state on waking).

- ***Timing***: Napping is most effective when used to bridge circadian "dead zones", for most, this lands in the hours after a night shift but before the body's drive for restorative sleep peaks. Avoid naps within two hours of a planned main sleep episode to prevent interference.

- ***Duration***: A 10- to 30-minute nap is ideal for alertness and memory, with minimal risk of dropping into deep sleep (slow-wave), which can worsen inertia. Going much longer—especially 60 or 90 minutes—may help relieve deeper deficits but often leaves you fighting heavy grogginess upon waking. For most on rotating or night shifts, the 20–30 minute range is the best balance.
- ***Sleep inertia control***: To reduce sleep inertia, nap during periods of lower sleep pressure if possible (for example, before your main sleep window). Expose yourself to bright light or engage in light movement immediately after waking. Caffeine may help, but timing is critical: too late and it can disrupt later sleep.

Step-by-step: Creating a 30-minute re-entry nap protocol for rotating shifts

If you finish your shift wired, overtired, or simply not ready to sleep fully, a structured nap can serve as a helpful bridge. Use this targeted protocol to deploy a nap effectively:

1. ***Set your environment***: Block out light (eye mask, blackout shades), reduce noise (earplugs or soft background noise). Keep the area comfortably cool.
2. ***Set a timer for 25–30 minutes***: This protects you from sliding into deeper sleep cycles that are harder to shake off.

3. ***Pre-nap wind-down***: Spend 2–3 minutes doing gentle breathwork or stretching to cue relaxation and lower residual adrenaline.
4. ***Nap***: Lie down with the goal of resting, not necessarily sleeping. Allow your body to disengage; shallow dozing is still restorative.
5. ***Gentle wake***: Use a non-jarring alarm. Upon waking, sit up slowly and expose yourself to light—open curtains or step outside if possible.
6. ***Quick reactivation***: Try light movement, such as standing, stretching, or brief walking, to shake off grogginess. Splash your face with cold water if inertia is strong.
7. ***Assess***: Notice if you feel more alert or if grogginess persists. If so, proceed to your longer sleep window soon rather than pushing through.

Checklist: Signs you need a nap vs. a full sleep episode

Distinguishing when to use a nap as opposed to a full sleep period matters for recovery and performance. Consider the following cues:

- ☐ Indicators for a nap:
- ☐ Mild to moderate fatigue but not overwhelming sleepiness.
- ☐ You have at least a few hours before your main sleep window.

- ☐ Cognitive "fuzziness" or slowed reaction time, but you're able to complete basic tasks.
- ☐ You need to be functional for a short drive or quick errand before real sleep.
- ☐ Indicators for a full sleep episode:
- ☐ Intense drowsiness that feels unmanageable.
- ☐ Microsleeps (brief, unintentional "nod offs").
- ☐ Trouble forming coherent thoughts or sentences.
- ☐ You have two or more hours available and little risk of interruption.
- ☐ Troubleshooting: When napping disrupts rather than helps after night shifts

Not every nap leads to improved function. Sometimes, they backfire, delaying or fragmenting your main sleep block, or leaving you groggier than before. Troubleshoot with these targeted adjustments:

- ***Napping too late***: If you nap within 60–90 minutes of your planned full daytime sleep, you may find falling asleep later much tougher.
- ***Nap too long***: Going past 30 minutes can drag you into slow-wave sleep, where waking is harder and effects linger.
- ***Chronic nap-dependency***: Overreliance on repeated naps during the day may signal you're not getting enough consolidated sleep. Aim to prioritize your main sleep episode whenever you can.

- ***Persistent sleep inertia***: If you wake from a short nap still severely foggy, experiment with briefer naps (10–20 min) and couple wake-ups with strong daylight exposure and movement.
- ***Trouble napping at all***: High adrenaline states can make it impossible to settle. In this case, skip the nap and try a physical decompression (such as a walk or shower), followed by your sleep routine.

Examples of re-entry routines: Bath, brief walk, daylight exposure

Not everyone can nap effectively, or you may find you need an alternative on particularly restless mornings. Re-entry routines can help reset your body and mind, especially if you're transitioning from work's intensity straight into the recovery window.

Three re-entry strategies that support sleep, mood, and alertness:

1. ***Warm bath or shower***: Immersion in warm water relaxes muscles and helps cue a drop in core body temperature, setting you up for sleep.
2. ***Brief outdoor walk***: Even a five-minute walk—especially if exposed to early daylight, can both clear residual stress and firm up your circadian timing. Daylight signals your brain it's time to wind down soon, paradoxical as it may feel after a night shift.

3. ***Deliberate light exposure***: If you're still edgy after your shift, intentionally exposing yourself to bright light for a short window (before your main sleep) can both cut grogginess and help "anchor" your biological clock, preventing it from drifting too far off course.

Pairing these routines with a strategic nap protocol (or using them when naps aren't possible) provides a flexible buffer, helping transition your body from emergency mode toward genuine rest.

In sum, leveraging short, well-timed naps and tailored re-entry rituals gives you more control over the unpredictable aftermath of night work. Rather than fighting your body's cues or relying solely on discipline, these strategies help align your recovery with how your real-life schedule and nervous system operate. Experiment with timing and sequence to find what fits best, and adapt as your shifts and recovery needs evolve.

Chapter 14: Signs You're Overdue for a Reset—and How to Intervene Early

Recognizing when you're overdue for a reset isn't always straightforward. Many night-shift clinicians are masters at suppressing discomfort, pushing through, and adapting "just one more time." Yet even the most resilient professionals hit a wall if warning signs are missed. This chapter arms you with a practical self-check, a clear intervention roadmap, and essential strategies to help you catch, and address burnout long before it becomes critical.

Spotting Red Flag Symptoms: Your Self-Check Tool

Catching the early signs of accumulating stress or exhaustion can mean the difference between a quick course correction and a lengthy recovery. Symptoms of burnout typically fall into three categories: physical, emotional, and behavioral. A quick self-check after a run of shifts (or any time you feel "off") can help you spot issues early.

Physical red flags include:

- Lingering headaches, stomach upsets, or muscle pain not explained by a single event
- Severe fatigue that doesn't ease with sleep or days off

- Noticeable changes in appetite or unintentional weight shifts
- Fuzzy thinking, frequent mistakes, or feeling "slowed down" physically

Emotional red flags often surface as:

- Heightened irritability, sudden anger, or feeling emotionally numb
- Frequent anxiety, tension, or a racing mind that won't settle—even when safe at home
- Loss of sense of purpose, dread about returning to work, or cynicism about your patients or team

Behavioral warning signs might include:

- Withdrawing from family or colleagues; skipping usual check-ins
- Reduced motivation even for self-care basics (showering, meal prep)
- Increased reliance on caffeine, sugar, alcohol, or other quick fixes
- Poor attention to safety steps at work or in daily life

If these symptoms pop up regularly or cluster together, treat them as a signal: your body and mind need a reset, not more pushing.

Three-Pronged Intervention: Immediate, Short-Term, and Long-Term Steps

When you detect warning signs, taking prompt and layered action works best. Here's a three-stage approach you can implement right away.

1. **Immediate: Interrupt and Stabilize**
    - Pause and acknowledge what you're feeling. Taking just sixty seconds to label your state—frustrated, overwhelmed, exhausted—activates self-awareness and helps break autopilot.
    - If you're at work and acutely overwhelmed (shaky, teary, or blank), step away if possible: a quick bathroom visit, splash of cold water, or focused breathwork (such as box breathing) can interrupt mounting distress.
    - Communicate your state to a trusted peer, supervisor, or family member if possible. Even briefly naming it (text, voice note) opens the door to support and accountability.

2. **Short-term: Downshift and Reset**
    - After your shift, structure a deliberate "reset window"—even ten minutes away from all work-related messages or noise can make a difference.

- Use your wind-down protocol: gentle movement, guided audio, or environmental cues that signal you're off-duty. Don't default to scrolling or numbing with distractions.
- Prioritize adequate sleep, nutrition, and hydration over everything else for the next 24 hours. Skipping these in the short term only extends recovery time.

3. **Long-term: Adjust and Safeguard**
   - If you've noticed a pattern of symptoms, take stock of your routines. Is your recovery protocol robust, or are rest and reset consistently getting sidelined?
   - Integrate non-negotiable recovery habits, protected sleep time, planned social connection, and meaningful wind-downs, into your schedule.
   - Regularly review your workload and boundaries. Consider if a schedule change, shift swap, or temporary workload reduction is realistic or needed. Decision Points: When to Seek Additional Support

Some warning signs call for more than self-management. Use the following criteria to decide if it's time to reach out:

- ***Persistent***: Symptoms last more than two weeks, or recur after even dedicated reset efforts.

- ***Impairing***: You consistently struggle to function at work or at home, or make mistakes you wouldn't normally make.
- ***Escalating***: You notice serious shifts, panic attacks, feeling hopeless, thoughts of self-harm, or severe detachment.
- ***Unmanageable***: Recovery steps no longer help, or you dread returning to every shift.

At this point, it's appropriate and necessary to involve others. Consider these options:

- ***Occupational health or employee assistance resources***: Many hospitals offer burnout intervention, counseling, or phased return-to-work plans.
- ***Peer support groups specific to clinicians or EMS***: Discussing challenges with others who share your schedule and pressures can be validating and resourceful.
- ***Mental health professionals***: Access a counselor or therapist experienced in working with healthcare professionals and shift workers.

If in doubt, err on the side of early outreach rather than later, intervening sooner reduces harm for you, your patients, and your team.

Printable: Crisis Interruption and Self-Triage Plan

Keep a one-page reference (either digital or paper) for moments of overwhelm. Here's a simple framework:

- ***Pause and self-check***: What am I feeling physically, emotionally, and behaviorally? Rate your distress 1–10.
- ***Interrupt***: Use a rapid technique (such as splash cold water, breathwork, checking in with a peer, or stepping into a quiet space).
- ***Reset minimum***: Commit to one small, positive action—hydrate, eat something nourishing, sit down in silence for five minutes, or do basic stretching.
- ***Escalate if needed***: If relief isn't noticeable within 15–30 minutes, and distress remains high (above a 7/10), seek support, call a colleague, supervisor, or professional helpline.

Customize this list with actions or contacts that fit your real work environment, so it's actionable when you most need it.

Pitfalls: The Dangers of Ignoring Early Signs

A common trap for high-performing clinicians is the belief that "toughing it out" is a mark of professionalism. Unfortunately, ignoring subtle red flags allows exhaustion to harden into chronic burnout, a state far harder to reverse.

Key mistakes include:

- Downplaying or normalizing persistent symptoms ("everyone feels this tired")
- Dismissing emotional numbing or irritability as standard "night-shifter mood"
- Delaying intervention until problems escalate, requiring extended leave or more invasive solutions

Remember, early action is not a sign of weakness. It's an investment in your long-term capability and well-being—and it helps prevent costly errors that put patients and colleagues at risk.

In summary, noticing and acting on even mild warning signs protects both career longevity and personal health. Layer your interventions, keep self-check tools close at hand, and treat early resets as core clinical skills—not optional extras. By intervening before stress takes over, you set yourself up for sustained resilience and effectiveness across your unique shiftwork reality.

References and Helpful Links

Following up on early identification and intervention techniques, this final chapter compiles the evidence, expert guidance, and practical resources behind the protocols and tools presented throughout the guide. Whether you want to explore the science further, update your practice, or access ongoing support, these references will serve as a reliable foundation.

Curated Peer-Reviewed Studies on Shift Work, Fatigue, and Sleep Intervention

For clinicians, understanding the concrete risks and solutions behind night-shift work starts with research. The following peer-reviewed articles were selected for their methodological rigor and direct relevance to night-shift clinical environments:

Åkerstedt, T. (2003). Shift work and disturbed sleep/wakefulness. Occupational Medicine, 53(2), 89–94. Explores circadian misalignment and sleep challenges unique to rotating and night-shift workers.

Rajaratnam, S.M.W., & Arendt, J. (2001). Health in a 24-h society. The Lancet, 358(9286), 999–1005. Addresses long-term health effects of persistent circadian disruption and fatigue.

Taylor, D.J., & Bramoweth, A.D. (2010). Patterns and consequences of inadequate sleep in healthcare workers. Sleep Medicine Clinics, 5(1), 43–54. Summarizes sleep deficit patterns and patient safety implications.

Barger, L.K. et al. (2006). Impact of extended-duration shifts on medical errors. New

England Journal of Medicine, 352(2), 125–134. A pivotal study on fatigue-driven error rates in hospital staff.

Kecklund, G., & Axelsson, J. (2016). Health consequences of shift work and insufficient sleep. BMJ, 355, i5210. Reviews physiological and cognitive effects in high-responsibility professions.

Neil-Sztramko, S.E. et al. (2014). Effect of workplace-based sleep education on shift worker sleep and alertness. Scandinavian Journal of Work, Environment & Health, 40(6), 593–603. Assesses educational interventions to improve post-shift recovery.

For a deeper understanding, consider reviewing meta-analyses synthesizing dozens of studies, such as:

Flo, E. et al. (2012). Shift work disorder in nurses: Prevalence and consequences. A systematic review. Sleep and Biological Rhythms, 10(4), 231-239.

Authoritative Guidelines from Major Organizations

The following organizations set evidence-based standards and recommendations highly relevant to clinicians navigating shift work. They offer up-to-date frameworks for both individual workers and institutions.

Centers for Disease Control and Prevention (CDC): "NIOSH Training for Nurses on Shift Work and Long Work Hours." This comprehensive resource details risk patterns, practical mitigations, and organizational responsibilities. [Link: www.cdc.gov/niosh/work-hour-training-for-nurses]

National Institute for Occupational Safety and Health (NIOSH): NIOSH's "Plain Language About Shiftwork" reference summarizes risks and recommended adaptations for healthcare workers across settings.

American Academy of Sleep Medicine (AASM): Clinical Practice Guidelines for shift work disorder and sleep maintenance offer practical, stepwise recommendations for clinicians.

Sleep Foundation: "Shift Work Sleep Disorder" overview. Covers causes, symptoms, and validated treatment options with an accessible, clinician-friendly format.

Society for Occupational Medicine (SOM): Detailed position statements on workplace fatigue and recommended preventive policies.

Key Books and Meta-Analyses on Nervous System Regulation in Clinicians

Insights into effective reset routines and nervous system support are drawn from inter-professional research and clinical handbooks. The following titles provide foundational knowledge:

"Why We Sleep" by Matthew Walker, PhD. Provides clarity on the mechanics and importance of restorative rest, relevant for any night-shift worker.

"The Body Keeps the Score" by Bessel van der Kolk, MD. While focused on trauma, this book delves into nervous system regulation methods beneficial for clinicians with chronic stress.

"Rest: Why You Get More Done When You Work Less" by Alex Soojung-Kim Pang. A practical guide to developing micro-restorative habits, including evidence-based recovery protocols.

For neuroscience-driven approaches tailored to those in high-pressure environments:

McEwen, B.S. (2006). Sleep deprivation as a neurobiologic and physiologic stressor:

Allostasis and allostatic load. Metabolism, 55, S20-S23.

Fallis, W.M. et al. (2011). Strategies to promote sleep in shift workers: Meta-analysis.

Journal of Advanced Nursing, 67(5), 929-940.

Resources for Further Reading and Support

As you encounter new challenges, these resources can help deepen your knowledge or connect you with expert guidance—a crucial step if chronic fatigue or stress persists.

Sleep Research Society (www.sleepresearchsociety.org): Offers up-to-date research updates, educational webinars, and networking opportunities for health professionals interested in sleep science.

National Sleep Foundation (www.sleepfoundation.org): In-depth resources on sleep hygiene, workplace fatigue, and clinical assessment tools.

International Association for the Study of Pain (IASP) "Sleep & Pain" Toolkit: Particularly helpful for clinicians experiencing pain-related sleep disruption.

Employee Assistance Programs (EAP): Most hospital or EMS employers offer free, confidential access to counseling, peer support, and stress management workshops. If you're overwhelmed or suspect burnout, this is a critical entry point for help.

Local medical libraries and institutional repositories are also worthwhile sources for reviewing the latest clinical guidelines and workplace mental health literature.

Citation of Worksheets, Checklists, and Protocols

Every worksheet, checklist, and protocol featured in this guide is either directly sourced from or adapted in line with published scientific literature and clinical best practice. Key sources include:

Fatigue self-check and symptom trackers: Adapted from CDC/NIOSH shift work fatigue surveillance templates.

Wind-down and breathwork protocols: Based on AASM and Sleep Foundation guidance for acute nervous system decompression.

Environmental sleep hygiene checklists: Synthesized from NIOSH, Sleep Foundation, and peer-reviewed occupational sleep studies.

Nutrition and caffeine tracking worksheets: Informed by research in BMJ and Sleep

Medicine Clinics, corroborated with National Sleep Foundation dietary recommendations.

Transition rituals and micro-connection templates: Developed by synthesizing strategies from McEwen (allostatic load) and van der Kolk (nervous system reset modalities), with practical adaptations from occupational health education.

Permission to reproduce or modify these materials for personal use is granted with citation to this guide and source references above.

Closing Notes

Access to high-quality reference material isn't just academic—it ensures that your after-shift reset routines are safe, effective, and defensible. Leverage these studies, guidelines, and tools as both a foundation and a springboard for making your recovery practices more resilient. If in doubt or facing persistent symptoms, use these resources to seek targeted support and keep your well-being a priority as your career evolves.

Conclusion: Consolidating Your New-Found Reset Superpowers

You now have a robust set of evidence-based strategies for winding down after a night shift, regulating your nervous system, and cultivating restorative sleep, each tailored for the specific realities faced by clinicians working through the night. These tools aren't generic wellness tips or abstract science. They're actionable, time-efficient routines you can deploy at the end of even the most demanding shift: structured wind-down protocols, physical and breathwork resets, quick environment modifications, and practical approaches to managing mental replay and social interactions.

Rather than expecting instant perfection or a total overhaul, focus on selective, meaningful changes. Use the toolkit as a flexible resource rather than a rigid rulebook. Your energy levels, living situation, and the unpredictable nature of clinical work will constantly shape what's possible after any given shift. Instead of searching for a single ultimate reset routine, experiment with different combinations from this guide. You might find that a basic breathwork protocol and blackout curtain upgrade provide outsized returns, or maybe integrating a brief transition ritual and one nutrition tweak makes the biggest difference. The most effective routines will often be the simplest, adapted to your current constraints and needs.

Remember, sustainable improvement is usually the result of gradual integration rather than sweeping transformation. If adding multiple new habits feels daunting, zero in on just one or two changes that seem manageable right now. This could mean setting up your sleep space before leaving for work, or trying a 10-minute wind-down routine in the car before you head home. Even these smallest shifts have measurable impacts, on your recovery speed, cognitive sharpness, and the risk of chronic fatigue or safety errors. Incremental progress, revisited regularly, pays the greatest dividends over time.

Give yourself permission to refine and cycle through tools as your shifts, roles, and personal life evolve. What works best after a string of high-adrenaline emergencies may differ from what you need after a quieter night. Keep notes, use the checklists, and don't hesitate to switch up your approach if a habit starts to lose its effect. Treat your recovery process as dynamic adaptation is a core part of resilience for night-shift professionals.

Above all, recognize that protecting your ability to reset isn't simply a bonus; it's a baseline requirement for both personal well-being and professional safety. The cost of ignoring after-shift recovery has been clearly mapped in research, personal testimonials, and institutional guidelines referenced here. You now have both the science and step-by-step instructions to make targeted changes.

Consolidating your reset superpowers comes down to ongoing experimentation, honest self-assessment, and embracing small, consistent adjustments. Integrate just a handful of these tools, tailored to your work and life demands, and the impact on your health, performance, and career longevity will be real and lasting. Your recovery matters, for you, for your patients, and for everyone who counts on your skill and steadiness day after day.

www.ingramcontent.com/pod-product-compliance
Lightning Source LLC
LaVergne TN
LVHW022009200926
848481LV00007B/2305
* 9 7 9 8 2 9 5 5 8 0 0 6 2 *